ARTHRITIS DIET HANDBOOK

A COMPLETE DIET PLAN FOR ARTHRITIS

KEATON LOWE

Table of Contents

CHAPTER 1

The diet for arthritis

Over 150 different conditions fall under the umbrella term "arthritis." Because they affect the muscles, bones, and joints, we should use the term musculoskeletal conditions instead.

Everyone can benefit from eating well to keep their health in check, even if there isn't a "miracle food" to cure arthritis or other musculoskeletal conditions.

Dietary changes may be beneficial in the treatment of some conditions. When it comes to examples:

Omega-3 fats, found in oily fish like sardines and salmon, may help people with inflammatory conditions like rheumatoid arthritis.

Purine-rich foods like offal, shellfish and beer should be avoided by people with gout (a type of arthritis) and water should be consumed frequently.

When you eat a wide variety of nutritious foods, your body functions optimally. All the vitamins, minerals, antioxidants, and other nutrients your body needs can be found in a well-balanced diet.

Incorporate fish, nuts, olive oil and plenty of fruits and vegetables into your diet to reap the health benefits of the Mediterranean diet. Additionally, eating a well-balanced diet and drinking plenty of fluids can improve your energy levels and help you maintain a healthy weight, which may alleviate your symptoms.

Before making any major changes to your diet, always consult with your doctor or dietitian. It's possible that you're restricting your food intake or taking too many products (like mineral supplements) that have no effect on your condition. Your medication may interact with some supplements.

Weight loss and arthritis go hand in hand.

If you have arthritis in your hips, knees, feet, or spine, the extra weight on your joints may be aggravating your symptoms of obesity-related arthritis. Being overweight is also associated with an increased risk of osteoarthritis.

People with arthritis may find it difficult to exercise because of their pain or stiffness. See a doctor, dietitian, or other health care professional for information and advice..

Researchers have discovered that foods high in omega-3 fats help reduce inflammation in some types of arthritis, including rheumatoid arthritis. Although these effects are modest in comparison to medication, they are free of side effects and may have additional health benefits such as a decreased risk of heart disease.

Omega-3-rich foods include:

oily fish like salmon and sardines •

flaxseed oil (also known as linseed) and linseeds

oil made from rapeseed or canola

• walnuts

Foods such as margarine and eggs that have been enriched with omega-3s

Fish oil supplements, for example

Contrary to popular belief, fish oils are not to be confused with fish liver oils (such as cod liver oil and halibut liver oil). Additionally, fish liver oils are a good source of vitamin A. Supplementing with excessive amounts of vitamin A can result in serious health complications. Before taking any supplements, check with your doctor to make sure you're getting the right dosage.

CHAPTER 2

Rheumatoid arthritis (RA) is a painful condition in which crystals of uric acid (a naturally occurring waste product) build up in a joint, usually the big toe.

Small dietary changes may help lower uric acid levels, which may reduce the likelihood of future gout attacks. Among the modifications are:

restricting or abstaining from drinking

- refraining from excessive drinking

Offal meats, such as liver and kidney are to be avoided or restricted if possible

limit or avoid shellfish like prawns and scallops, for example

seafood such as herrings and sardines, as well as mackerel and anchovies products that contain yeast, such as beer and Vegemite, should be restricted or avoided

taking in lots of fluids

• consuming a diet rich in fresh fruits and vegetables

• Avoiding fasting or a crash-diet regimen

• ensuring that you don't regularly overeat.

Changing your diet in a healthy way can be made easier if you work with a doctor or a dietitian.

The underlying cause of gout, excess uric acid in the blood, cannot be addressed by dietary changes alone. Gout medications, if prescribed by your doctor, must be taken as prescribed.

Arthritis and glucosamine/chondroitin

Glucosamine and chondroitin are popular supplements, but there is little evidence to support their use in the treatment of arthritis.

In some studies, people with osteoarthritis who take either glucosamine sulphate or chondroitin may notice a reduction in pain. This supplement does not appear to help with any other type of arthritis.

Chondroitin and glucosamine have been shown to interact with warfarin, so they must be taken only under the guidance of a physician.

Evidence linking a healthy diet to a reduced risk of arthritis

Avoiding certain foods and taking gout medication may help prevent gout attacks in people with gout.

But there is no evidence that avoiding certain foods can help alleviate or improve other forms of arthritis.

Arthritis and other musculoskeletal conditions aren't caused or aggravated by the following foods, according to scientific evidence.

• foods with a high acid content, such as lemons, limes, and oranges

The so-called "nightshade" family of vegetables and fruits includes:

• milk products.

The absence of these foods can lead to a host of other health issues, so it's important to eat them.

In some cases, eliminating foods that a person is intolerant to can help them feel better in the long run. Exactly what effect this has on arthritis symptoms, on the other hand, remains a mystery. Consult a dietitian before excluding any foods from your diet to ensure that you're not omitting vital nutrients.

Suggestions for Arthritis Diet Management

If you have arthritis, here are some suggestions for a healthy diet:

It is imperative that you consume an array of nutrients in a well-balanced diet in order to reap the many health benefits that come with it.

Variety of fruits and vegetables, as well as a wide variety of protein foods (e.g. milk), nuts, pulses, cereals, etc. Maintaining a healthy weight and general well-being will be aided by this.

Take in plenty of omega-3 fatty acids in the form of oils like canola or flax seed or foods that have been fortified with omega-3 fatty acids in your diet (for example, eggs or margarine) drinking plenty of water is essential to good health

• eat a diet rich in calcium to prevent osteoporosis in old age

Obesity puts additional strain on joints, particularly those that bear weight, such as the knees and hips.

It may be helpful to keep track of your food intake and symptoms in a food diary if you suspect a certain food is aggravating your condition. The food that is causing your symptoms might become apparent after a month. Find a doctor or a nutritionist to discuss this information with.

without consulting your doctor, don't eliminate entire food groups from your diet, such as dairy products, without first consulting your doctor.

It is important to be aware that the symptoms of arthritis, particularly inflammatory types, can change without any apparent reason. Any improvement in your symptoms isn't necessarily the result of your diet or what you eat. Be sure to follow the advice of your doctor or other health care professional.

consult with a doctor or a nutritionist if you need help. Arthritis and diet are the subject of much debate on the internet and in the media. Consult a specialist if you're stuck.

10 Foods That Help Arthritis Patients

If you suffer from arthritis, you are well aware of the debilitating effects it can have on your life.

CHAPTER 3

The term "arthritis" refers to a group of diseases characterized by inflammation, stiffness, and pain in the joints. People of all ages, genders, and ethnicities can be affected by it.

Osteoarthritis is a multifaceted disease. Overuse of joints can lead to osteoarthritis, one type of the disease. Rheumatoid arthritis, an autoimmune disease in which your immune system attacks your joints, is yet another type of arthritis to consider.

Fortunately, there are a number of foods that can reduce inflammation and alleviate some of the joint pain associated with arthritis.

Some 24% of those with rheumatoid arthritis reported that their diet had an impact on their symptoms, according to a survey conducted in 2012.

Fatty Fish #1

Omega-3 fatty acids, found in fatty fish like salmon, mackerel, sardines, and trout, have been shown to have powerful anti-inflammatory properties.

Fatty fish, lean fish, or lean meat were fed to 33 participants four times a week in one small study. Researchers found that those who consumed more fatty fish had lower levels of inflammation-related compounds after eight weeks of supplementation.

Supplementing with omega-3 fatty acids can reduce joint pain, morning stiffness, the number of pain-inducing joints, and pain-relieving medication use in patients with RA, according to an analysis of 17 studies.

Omega-3 fatty acids were also shown in a test tube study to reduce several osteoarthritis-related inflammatory markers.

Vitamin D, which is found in fish, can help prevent vitamin D deficiency. Multiple studies have linked rheumatoid arthritis to vitamin D deficiency, which may be a contributing factor in the disease's symptoms.

The anti-inflammatory properties of fatty fish are recommended by the American Heart Association to be included in your diet at least twice a week.

2. The flavor of garlic

Garlic has a slew of health benefits, including anti-inflammatory properties.

Garlic and its components have been found to have cancer-fighting properties in some laboratory studies. They also contain compounds that may reduce the risk of heart disease and Alzheimer's disease, among other things.

Studies have shown that garlic has anti-inflammatory properties that could reduce arthritis symptoms.

As a matter of fact, some studies have shown that garlic may enhance the function of certain immune cells in order to improve the immune system.

The diets of 1,082 twins were studied in a single study by researchers at Stanford University. In their study, they found that those who ate more garlic had a lower risk of developing hip osteoarthritis, likely due to the anti-inflammatory properties of the herb.

Some of the inflammatory markers associated with arthritis can be reduced by a specific component in garlic, according to another test-tube study.

Ginger is number three on our list.

Ginger, in addition to enhancing the flavor of teas, soups, and desserts, may also help alleviate the pain and discomfort of arthritis sufferers.

Ginger extract was tested on 261 patients with knee osteoarthritis in a 2001 study. Sixty-three percent of participants reported a decrease in knee pain after six weeks.

Ginger and its constituents have also been shown in a test tube study to inhibit the production of substances in the body that promote inflammation.

Another study found that treating rats with ginger extract reduced the levels of a specific inflammatory marker linked to the development of arthritis.

Ginger is number three on our list.

Ginger, in addition to enhancing the flavor of teas, soups, and desserts, may also help alleviate the pain and discomfort of arthritis sufferers.

Ginger extract was tested on 261 patients with knee osteoarthritis in a 2001 study. Six weeks later, 63% of participants reported less pain in their knees.

Ginger and its components were also found to inhibit the production of substances that promote inflammation in the body in a test-tube study.

Researchers found that ginger extract reduced levels of an

inflammation marker linked to arthritis in rats.

Broccoli is number four.

Broccoli is widely recognized as one of the healthiest vegetables available. As a matter of fact, it may even reduce inflammation.

The consumption of cruciferous vegetables like broccoli was linked to lower levels of inflammatory markers, according to one study that examined the diets of 1,005 women.

Arthritis symptoms may be alleviated by consuming broccoli, which contains important components.

Broccoli, for example, contains a compound called sulforaphane. Rheumatoid arthritis is caused by a type of cell that is blocked by it in test-tube studies.

Animal studies have shown that sulforaphane can lessen

inflammatory markers that contribute to arthritis, as well.

More research in humans and animals is required, but these results from the test tube and animal studies show that the compounds in broccoli may help reduce arthritis symptoms.

CHAPTER 4

Walnuts are number five on our list.

Inflammation in the joints can be reduced by eating walnuts, which are high in nutrients and contain compounds that may reduce inflammation.

A review of 13 studies found a link between walnut

consumption and lower inflammation markers.

The omega-3 fatty acids found in walnuts, in particular, have been shown to reduce arthritis symptoms.

Olive oil or omega-3 fatty acid supplementation was given to 90 patients with rheumatoid arthritis in a single clinical trial.

Patients who received omega-3 fatty acids had lower levels of pain and reduced their use of arthritis medications compared to those who received olive oil.

Research on omega-3 fatty acids and arthritis has been largely focused on the general effects of omega-3 fatty acids. To learn more about the effects of walnuts in particular, more research is needed.

Berries are number six.

Antioxidants, vitamins, and minerals abound in berries, which may explain in part why they're so effective at reducing inflammation.

In a study of 38,176 women, those who ate at least two servings of strawberries per week were 14 percent less likely to have an elevated level of inflammatory markers in the blood.

Berries are also high in quercetin and rutin, two plant compounds with a slew of health benefits.

Quercetin was found to inhibit some of the inflammatory processes linked to arthritis in a test tube study.

Other studies have shown that quercetin and rutin supplements can help reduce inflammation in arthritis.

Fortunately, a wide variety of berries are available if you'd like to take advantage of these impressive health benefits. You can satisfy your sweet tooth while getting plenty of arthritis-fighting nutrients from strawberries, blackberries, and blueberries.

Spinach is number seven.

Spinach, a leafy green, is rich in nutrients and may be able to help reduce arthritis-related inflammation.

Fruits and vegetables have been linked to lower inflammation levels in numerous studies.

Antioxidants and anti-inflammatory plant compounds abound in spinach, making it an excellent anti-inflammatory food.

Rheumatoid arthritis-related inflammatory mediators can be lessened by spinach's high concentration of the antioxidant kaempferol

CHAPTER 5

Kaempferol has been shown to reduce inflammation and slow the progression of osteoarthritis in a 2017 study on arthritic cartilage cells.

Research into the effects of spinach and its constituents on arthritis sufferers is still needed.

Spinach is a vegetable

antioxidants, such as kaempferol, are abundant in Test-tube research has shown that

Inflammation and the progression of disease can be reduced by kaempferol

osteoarthritis.

Grapes

In addition to being high in antioxidants and anti-inflammatory properties, grapes are packed with nutrients.

At the beginning of the study, 24 men were given either 1.5 cups (252 grams) of fresh grapes or a placebo each day for three weeks. Inflammatory markers in the blood were reduced by the use of grape powder.

A number of compounds found in grapes have been shown to be helpful in the treatment of rheumatoid arthritis. Resveratrol, an antioxidant found in the skin of grapes, is one such example.

According to one study, resveratrol may help prevent arthritis-related joint thickening by preventing the formation of rheumatoid arthritis cells in test tubes.

Proanthocyanidin, another plant compound found in grapes, has been shown to have promising anti-arthritic effects. Grape seed proanthocyanidin extract, for example, was found to reduce inflammation in a test-tube study.

Keep in mind that these studies were conducted in a laboratory setting with much higher concentrations of antioxidants than you would find in a typical serving.

More research is needed to see if these findings apply to people.

Nuts and Seeds

Olive oil, which is known for its anti-inflammatory properties, may help alleviate the symptoms of arthritis.

Extra-virgin olive oil was fed to mice for six weeks in one study. As a result, the progression of arthritis was slowed, joint swelling was reduced, cartilage degradation was slowed, and inflammation was reduced.

An olive oil capsule or fish oil capsule was given to 49 people with rheumatoid arthritis every day for 24 weeks in another study.

A specific inflammatory marker's levels decreased in both groups by the end of the study, but in the olive oil group by 38.5 percent and in the fish oil group by 40–55 percent.

Olive oil consumption was linked to a lower risk of developing rheumatoid arthritis, according to another study, which looked at the diets of 333 people with and without the disease.

Olive oil and other healthy fats in your diet can have a positive impact on your health and may even reduce your arthritis symptoms, despite the fact that more research is needed.

ten. Cherry Juice with Tartness

The Prunus cerasus tree's fruit, tart cherry juice, is becoming an increasingly popular beverage.

Many nutrients and health benefits can be found in this powerful juice, including the possibility of easing the pain associated with rheumatoid arthritis (RA).

Every day for six weeks, 58 participants were given either a placebo or two 8-ounce (237 ml) bottles of tart cherry juice.

It was found that tart cherry juice reduced symptoms of

osteoarthritis and decreased inflammation.

In another study, women with osteoarthritis who drank tart cherry juice for three weeks saw a decrease in inflammatory markers.

Keep an eye out for unsweetened tart cherry juice to avoid consuming unnecessary sugar.

A daily serving of unsweetened tart cherry juice may help alleviate some of the symptoms of arthritis in combination with a healthy diet and other arthritis-fighting foods.

The Verdict

Clearly, diet can have a significant impact on the severity and symptoms of arthritis.

Thanks to their powerful components, many food items have the potential to reduce inflammation and arthritis pain while also improving general wellbeing.

Some of the symptoms of arthritis may be alleviated by eating a healthy diet rich in healthy fats, some fatty fish, and a wide variety of fruits and vegetables, in addition to conventional treatments.

THE END